TYPE 2 DIABETES CODE:

A GUIDE ON MANAGING IT AND LIVING WELL

DISCLAIMER

The information contained in this resource is general in nature and for informative purposes only.

The Author assumes no responsibility whatsoever, under any circumstances, for any actions taken as a result of the information contained herein.

You are required to seek professional help if needed.

Before this document is duplicated or reproduced in any manner, the publisher's consent must be gained. Therefore, the contents within can neither be stored electronically, transferred, nor kept in a database.

Neither in Part nor full can the document be copied, scanned, faxed, or retained without approval from the publisher or creator.

Preface

The shelves of bookstores are filled with many fine books on Diabetes and Type 2 Diabetes. Why another one? I believe there is always a need for simple truths – no matter how often they are told

The issue of Type 2 Diabetes has become a worrisome one to a lot of people suffering from this.

If by reading this book, a person can say" Wow, now I get it. I see something that could really help me*, then my purpose as an author has been fulfilled.

One of the greatest motivations in my own life is to see someone who has been dealing with a particular issue experience remarkable life change.

If I can help someone understand and apply the tips that he or she otherwise would have missed, then creating this book will have one of the most rewarding experience of my life.

LEO CHAMBERS

INTRODUCTION

The prevalence of type 2 diabetes has reached alarming levels worldwide, making it a significant public health concern. With the increasing number of individuals affected by this chronic condition, there is a pressing need for comprehensive understanding and effective management strategies. This book aims to provide a comprehensive overview of type 2 diabetes, equipping readers with the knowledge and tools necessary to navigate this complex condition.

In this introductory section, we will define and explain type 2 diabetes, shedding light on its impact and significance. Type 2 diabetes is a metabolic disorder characterized by high blood sugar levels resulting from insulin resistance and impaired glucose metabolism. Unlike type 1 diabetes, which is an autoimmune condition, type 2 diabetes is often associated with lifestyle factors such as poor diet, sedentary behavior, and obesity.

The prevalence of type 2 diabetes has been steadily rising, affecting millions of individuals worldwide. Its consequences extend beyond the physical realm, as it can lead to various complications, including cardiovascular diseases, kidney problems, and nerve damage. Therefore, understanding and effectively managing type 2 diabetes is crucial for maintaining overall health and well-being.

Throughout this book, we will delve into the underlying causes of type 2 diabetes, exploring the physiological mechanisms that contribute to insulin resistance and impaired glucose metabolism. We will also discuss the diagnostic criteria and classification of type 2 diabetes, enabling readers to better understand their own condition or that of their loved ones.

Managing type 2 diabetes requires a multifaceted approach, encompassing lifestyle modifications, medication regimens, and self-care practices. In subsequent chapters, we will explore these aspects in detail, providing practical guidance on healthy eating, regular physical activity, weight management, and medication options. Additionally, we will emphasize the importance of monitoring blood glucose levels, regular check-ups, and preventive measures to minimize the risk of complications.

Living with type 2 diabetes can present unique challenges, both physically and emotionally. Therefore, we will address the psychological and emotional aspects of diabetes, offering strategies for coping and maintaining a positive mindset. Furthermore, we will highlight the support systems and resources available to individuals with diabetes, fostering a sense of community and empowerment.

As research in the field of diabetes continues to evolve, we will also discuss future directions and potential breakthroughs. Advances in diabetes management and treatment options hold promise for improved outcomes and quality of life for those living with type 2 diabetes. Staying informed and educated about these developments is essential for individuals and healthcare professionals alike.

In conclusion, this book aims to provide a comprehensive guide to understanding and managing type 2 diabetes. By equipping readers with knowledge, practical strategies, and a supportive framework, we hope to empower individuals to take control of their diabetes journey and lead healthy, fulfilling lives. Let us embark on this journey together, as we navigate the complexities of type 2 diabetes and strive for optimal well-being.

Table of Contents

Chapter 1
Understanding The Diabetes Malady And Types

It is crucial to understand the severe consequences that diabetes can have on a person's health. This condition is a leading cause of various ailments such as blindness, kidney failure, heart attacks, stroke, and lower limb amputation.

The impact of diabetes on mortality rates is also alarming. Between 2000 and 2019, there was a noticeable 3% increase in diabetes mortality rates across different age groups. Fortunately, there are various ways to prevent or delay the onset of type 2 diabetes. Adopting a healthy diet, engaging in regular physical activity, maintaining a normal body weight, and avoiding tobacco use are all effective measures to decrease the risk of developing this condition.

Moreover, it is crucial to recognize that diabetes can be treated, and its associated complications can be avoided or delayed. Managing diabetes involves a multifaceted approach, which includes dietary modifications, engaging in regular physical activity, taking prescribed medication, and undergoing consistent screening for potential complications.

In conclusion, the rise in diabetes cases globally is a concerning trend, particularly in low- and middle-income countries. The detrimental effects of diabetes on individuals' health and mortality rates cannot be underestimated. However, by implementing preventive measures and adopting appropriate treatment strategies, the burden of diabetes can be significantly reduced, ultimately improving the well-being of individuals affected by this condition.

In 2019 alone, diabetes and kidney disease resulting from diabetes were responsible for an estimated 2 million deaths worldwide. These statistics highlight the urgent need for effective prevention and management strategies.

There are several key facts to consider regarding diabetes. Firstly, the number of people affected by this condition has significantly increased over the years. In 1980, there were 108 million individuals with diabetes, but by 2014, this number had skyrocketed to 422 million. Interestingly, the prevalence of diabetes has been rising at a much faster rate in low- and middle-income countries compared to high-income countries.

Statistics reveal the widespread impact of diabetes on global health. In 2014, it was reported that 8.5% of adults aged 18 and above were affected by diabetes.

The year 2019 witnessed diabetes as the direct cause of 1.5 million deaths, with 48% of those deaths occurring before the age of 70. Additionally, diabetes was responsible for 460,000 deaths related to kidney disease, and approximately 20% of cardiovascular deaths were attributed to raised blood glucose levels.

There are two distinct types of diabetes: type 1 and type 2.

In type 1 diabetes, the pancreas ceases to produce insulin, while in type 2 diabetes, the body becomes resistant to normal or even high levels of insulin, eventually resulting in inadequate insulin production by the pancreas. Diabetes is a chronic condition that arises when the pancreas fails to produce an adequate amount of insulin or when the body is unable to effectively utilize the insulin it does produce.

Insulin plays a crucial role in regulating blood glucose levels. If diabetes is left uncontrolled, it can lead to hyperglycemia, which is characterized by elevated blood sugar levels. Over time, this can result in severe damage to various systems within the body, particularly the nerves and blood vessels.

From 2000 to 2019, there was a significant 3% increase in age-standardized mortality rates associated with diabetes. This increase was more pronounced in lower-middle-income countries, where the mortality rate due to diabetes rose by 13%.

Conversely, globally, the probability of dying from any of the four main noncommunicable diseases (cardiovascular diseases, cancer, chronic respiratory diseases, or diabetes) between the ages of 30 and 70 decreased by 22% during the same period.

Type 2 diabetes, also known as type 2 diabetes mellitus, is a condition that disrupts the body's ability to properly utilize glucose (sugar). It also affects the storage and processing of other forms of energy, such as fat. Every cell in the body relies on sugar for normal functioning, and insulin is the hormone responsible for facilitating the entry of sugar into cells. However, individuals with diabetes either have insufficient insulin or their bodies become unresponsive to its presence, leading to a buildup of sugar in the bloodstream. If left untreated, high blood sugar levels can give rise to various health complications.

In the United States, Canada, and Europe, the majority of individuals with diabetes, specifically around 90 percent, are diagnosed with type 2 diabetes. This particular form of diabetes is a chronic medical condition that necessitates constant monitoring and treatment throughout one's lifetime to maintain blood sugar levels as close to normal as possible.

Managing type 2 diabetes involves making significant lifestyle changes, including alterations to diet and exercise routines, as well as practicing self-care measures and potentially taking medications. Thankfully, these treatment methods have proven effective in controlling blood sugar levels and reducing the risk of developing complications associated with the condition.

This discussion aims to provide a comprehensive overview of type 2 diabetes. The impact of being diagnosed with this condition can be both alarming and overwhelming for individuals, as it raises numerous questions regarding its development, long-term health implications, and impact on daily life. It is natural to seek answers and guidance during this time, and healthcare professionals such as doctors or nurses are available to address these concerns and provide necessary information.

Additionally, they can offer valuable resources for both medical and psychological support, such as group classes, consultations with registered dietitians, social workers, or nurse educators, and access to educational materials like books, websites, or magazines that focus on diabetes management.

The initial period following a diabetes diagnosis is characterized by a rollercoaster of emotions for the majority of individuals. During this crucial time, it is essential for both you and your family to seize the opportunity to gather as much information as possible, enabling you to effectively manage your diabetes on a daily basis. This includes familiarizing yourself with tasks such as monitoring your blood sugar levels, attending medical appointments, and adhering to medication regimens. By embracing this learning phase, you can seamlessly incorporate these diabetes management practices into your routine.

The majority of individuals with diabetes are able to maintain an active lifestyle and partake in the same foods and activities as before their diagnosis. Having diabetes does not signify the end of indulging in treats like birthday cake, and most individuals with the condition are encouraged to engage in physical activity in various forms.

Symptoms of diabetes can manifest suddenly, but in the case of type 2 diabetes, they may appear mild and go unnoticed for several years. These symptoms include an excessive feeling of thirst, increased frequency of urination, blurred vision, fatigue, and unintentional weight loss.

However, the consequences of diabetes extend beyond these initial symptoms. Furthermore, diabetes often leads to nerve damage and poor blood flow in the feet, resulting in various foot problems. Many individuals with diabetes experience foot ulcers due to compromised nerve function and inadequate blood circulation. In severe cases, these ulcers can lead to the need for amputation.

Over time, diabetes can cause significant damage to blood vessels in vital organs such as the heart, eyes, kidneys, and nerves. This damage increases the risk of serious health problems such as heart attacks, strokes, and kidney failure. The eyes are particularly vulnerable to diabetes-related complications, as the condition can lead to permanent vision loss by damaging blood vessels in the eyes. Type 1 diabetes, previously referred to as insulin-dependent, juvenile, or childhood-onset diabetes, is characterized by the inadequate production of insulin. Consequently, individuals with this type of diabetes must administer insulin on a daily basis to manage their condition effectively.

Impaired glucose tolerance (IGT) and impaired fasting glycaemia (IFG) are intermediate conditions between normal blood glucose levels and diabetes. Individuals with IGT or IFG have a heightened risk of progressing to type 2 diabetes, although this progression is not inevitable.

Diagnosing diabetes early can be achieved through relatively inexpensive blood glucose testing. Individuals diagnosed with type 1 diabetes require insulin injections for their survival.

 Adopting a healthy lifestyle is one of the most crucial aspects of diabetes treatment. Some individuals with type 2 diabetes may also need to take medications, such as insulin injections or other prescribed drugs, to effectively manage their blood sugar level.

In the year 2017, the number of individuals diagnosed with type 1 diabetes reached a staggering 9 million. The majority of these individuals reside in high-income countries, although the exact cause and effective prevention methods for this condition remain unknown.

 Gestational diabetes is a temporary form of hyperglycemia that occurs during pregnancy. Although blood glucose values in gestational diabetes exceed normal levels, they fall below the diagnostic threshold for diabetes. Women with gestational diabetes face an elevated risk of complications during pregnancy and delivery. Additionally, both these women and their offspring are at a higher risk of developing type 2 diabetes in the future.

The diagnosis of gestational diabetes is made through prenatal screening rather than relying on reported symptoms. Fortunately, type 2 diabetes is often preventable. Several factors contribute to its development, such as being overweight, leading a sedentary lifestyle, and genetic predisposition. Detecting this condition early on is crucial to prevent its worst effects. Regular check-ups and blood tests with a healthcare provider are the most effective means of early detection.

It is noteworthy that over 95% of individuals with diabetes suffer from type 2 diabetes. Initially known as non-insulin dependent or adult-onset diabetes, this type was previously observed solely in adults.

However, it is now increasingly prevalent among children as well. The best approach to prevent or delay the onset of type 2 diabetes is through lifestyle modifications. Maintaining a healthy body weight, engaging in at least 30 minutes of moderate exercise per day, adhering to a nutritious diet while avoiding excessive sugar and saturated fat consumption, and abstaining from tobacco are all essential preventive measures.

The symptoms of type 2 diabetes can be mild and may take years to manifest. They may resemble those of type 1 diabetes but are typically less pronounced. Consequently, the diagnosis of this disease often occurs several years after its onset, by which time complications may have already arisen. Type 2 diabetes, on the other hand, directly affects the body's ability to utilize sugar (glucose) for energy. It hinders the proper functioning of insulin, which can result in elevated levels of blood sugar if left untreated. Over time, this particular type of diabetes can cause severe damage to various parts of the body, particularly the nerves and blood vessels.

In April 2021, WHO launched the Global Diabetes Compact, a global initiative aimed at improving diabetes prevention and care, with a focus on supporting low- and middle-income countries.

Additionally, the World Health Assembly adopted a resolution in May 2021 to strengthen the prevention and control of diabetes, and in May 2022, endorsed five global diabetes coverage and treatment targets to be achieved by 2030.

Furthermore, individuals with diabetes may require additional medical care to address the effects of the condition. This can include foot care to treat ulcers, screening and treatment for kidney disease, and regular eye exams to screen for retinopathy, which can lead to blindness.

The World Health Organization (WHO) is actively working to promote effective measures for the surveillance, prevention, and control of diabetes and its complications, particularly in low- and middle-income countries. This includes developing guidelines for diabetes prevention, establishing norms and standards for diagnosis and care, raising awareness about the global diabetes epidemic, and conducting surveillance of diabetes and its risk factors.

It is crucial to understand the complexities of type 2 diabetes and the various treatment options available to effectively manage the condition and reduce the risk of complications.

 There are several medications available to help manage type 2 diabetes, including metformin, sulfonylureas, and sodium-glucose co-transporters type 2 (SGLT-2) inhibitors. In addition to these medications, individuals with diabetes may also need to take medications to lower their blood pressure and statins to reduce the risk of complications.

Formerly referred to as adult-onset diabetes, type 2 diabetes can now develop in both children and adults, with older individuals being more commonly affected. The rise in childhood obesity has also led to an increase in cases of type 2 diabetes in younger populations. While there is no cure for this condition, managing it through weight loss, healthy eating, and physical activity can help control blood sugar levels. The primary causes of type 2 diabetes are insulin resistance in muscle, fat, and liver cells, as well as insufficient insulin production by the pancreas. The exact reasons for these issues are not completely understood, but being overweight and inactive are significant contributing factors.

 Treatment options may include lifestyle changes, medications, or insulin therapy if diet and exercise alone are not effective in controlling blood sugar levels. Type 2 diabetes is a chronic condition caused by issues with the body's regulation and utilization of sugar, also known as glucose. This leads to elevated blood sugar levels, which can lead to complications in the circulatory, nervous, and immune systems over time. In type 2 diabetes, the pancreas doesn't produce enough insulin and cells become resistant to insulin, resulting in inadequate sugar absorption.

Insulin, a hormone produced by the pancreas, plays a crucial role in regulating sugar levels in the body. When sugar is present in the bloodstream, the pancreas releases insulin, which allows sugar to enter cells.

As a result, the amount of sugar in the bloodstream decreases, leading to a decrease in insulin release. Glucose, the primary source of energy for cells, is obtained from food and the liver. With the help of insulin, glucose is absorbed into the bloodstream and enters cells. The liver stores and produces glucose, ensuring that the body maintains a healthy glucose level.

However, in individuals with type 2 diabetes, this process is disrupted. Instead of being absorbed into cells, sugar accumulates in the blood. Consequently, the pancreas releases more insulin as blood sugar levels rise. Over time, the insulin-producing cells in the pancreas become damaged, leading to insufficient insulin production.

Several risk factors contribute to the development of type 2 diabetes. Being overweight or obese increases the risk, as does the accumulation of fat in the abdominal area. Inactivity, family history of diabetes, certain racial and ethnic backgrounds, abnormal blood lipid levels, age, prediabetes, and a history of gestational diabetes or giving birth to a large baby are also associated with an increased risk.

The risk of type 2 diabetes is higher in men with a waist circumference above 40 inches (101.6 centimeters) and in women with a waist measurement above 35 inches (88.9 centimeters).

•   Inactivity. The less active a person is, the greater the risk. Physical activity helps control weight, uses up glucose as energy and makes cells more sensitive to insulin.

•   Family history. An individual's risk of type 2 diabetes increases if a parent or sibling has type 2 diabetes.

•   Race and ethnicity. Although it's unclear why, people of certain races and ethnicities — including Black, Hispanic, Native American and Asian people, and Pacific Islanders — are more likely to develop type 2 diabetes than white people are.

•   Blood lipid levels. An increased risk is associated with low levels of high-density lipoprotein (HDL) cholesterol — the "good" cholesterol — and high levels of triglycerides.

•   Age. The risk of type 2 diabetes increases with age, especially after age 35.

•   Prediabetes. Prediabetes is a condition in which the blood sugar level is higher than normal, but not high enough to be classified as diabetes.

Left untreated, prediabetes often progresses to type 2 diabetes.

- Pregnancy-related risks. The risk of developing type 2 diabetes is higher in people who had gestational diabetes when they were pregnant and in those who gave birth to a baby weighing more than 9 pounds (4 kilograms).

- Polycystic ovary syndrome. Having polycystic ovary syndrome — a condition characterized by irregular menstrual periods, excess hair growth and obesity — increases the risk of diabetes.

Chapter 2

Causes And Risk Factors of Type 2 Diabetes

Type 2 diabetes is believed to be caused by a combination of genetic and environmental factors.

The influence of genetics is evident, as many individuals with type 2 diabetes have a family member who also has the condition or other related health issues like high cholesterol, elevated triglyceride levels, hypertension, or obesity. The risk of developing type 2 diabetes is significantly higher for individuals with a first-degree relative, such as a sibling or child, with diabetes compared to those without a family history of the disease.

Moreover, certain ethnic groups, including those of Hispanic, African, and Asian descent, have a greater likelihood of developing type 2 diabetes.

However, it is important to note that environmental factors also play a crucial role in the development of this condition.

Unhealthy eating habits and a sedentary lifestyle contribute to weight gain, which significantly increases the risk of developing type 2 diabetes.

Therefore, it is essential to recognize the importance of both genetic and lifestyle factors in the onset of this disease.

During pregnancy, a minority of expectant mothers may develop a condition known as gestational diabetes, which is comparable to type 2 diabetes.

However, unlike type 2 diabetes, gestational diabetes typically disappears after childbirth. It is important to note that women who experience gestational diabetes are more likely to develop type 2 diabetes in the future.

There are several factors that can contribute to the development of type 2 diabetes.

One of the main causes is insulin resistance, where the body becomes resistant to the effects of insulin. This resistance prevents cells from effectively using insulin, leading to high blood sugar levels.

Additionally, beta cells in the pancreas, which are responsible for producing insulin, may not function properly in individuals with type 2 diabetes, resulting in reduced insulin production or impaired release.

 Another contributing factor is the accumulation of excess fat, particularly in the liver and pancreas, which can interfere with insulin production and secretion.

Chronic low-grade inflammation in the body can also impair insulin signaling and contribute to insulin resistance.

 Finally, hormonal imbalances, such as elevated levels of cortisol (the stress hormone) and reduced levels of adiponectin (a hormone involved in regulating glucose and fatty acid metabolism), can also play a role in the development of type 2 diabetes.

Furthermore, one of the major risk factors for type 2 diabetes is obesity. Being overweight or obese significantly increases the chances of developing the condition. Excessive body fat, particularly in the abdominal area, can lead to insulin resistance, further elevating the risk of diabetes.

It is crucial to understand that although these factors can heighten the likelihood of acquiring type 2 diabetes, they do not automatically mean that the condition will develop.

Making lifestyle changes, such as keeping a healthy weight, participating in consistent exercise, and following a well-rounded diet, can aid in decreasing the risk and effectively controlling the condition. It is also important to regularly schedule check-ups and screenings for early detection and timely intervention.

A sedentary lifestyle, characterized by a lack of physical activity, significantly raises the chances of developing type 2 diabetes. Engaging in regular exercise not only assists in managing a healthy weight but also enhances overall well-being.

Family history of type 2 diabetes can significantly heighten the chances of an individual developing this condition, as genetic factors play a crucial role in determining one's susceptibility to diabetes.

Furthermore, advancing age, particularly after reaching the age of 45, is closely associated with an increased risk of type 2 diabetes. This can be attributed to various factors including reduced physical activity levels, loss of muscle mass, and hormonal changes occurring within the body.

Additionally, certain ethnic groups, such as African Americans, Hispanics, Native Americans, and Asians, are more prone to developing type 2 diabetes compared to other ethnicities.

Lastly, women who have previously experienced gestational diabetes during pregnancy face an augmented risk of developing type 2 diabetes later in life.

Chapter 3

Symptoms and Diagnosis of Type 2 Diabetes

When symptoms do manifest, they can include various signs that indicate a disruption in the body's blood sugar regulation. Increased thirst, frequent urination, and heightened hunger are common symptoms that individuals may experience.

Additionally, unintended weight loss, fatigue, and blurred vision can also be indicators of type 2 diabetes. Other symptoms may include slow-healing sores, frequent infections, numbness or tingling in the hands or feet, and the presence of darkened skin in areas such as the armpits and neck.

In summary, the symptoms of type 2 diabetes can vary in their presentation and may develop slowly over time. It is important to be vigilant and seek medical attention if any symptoms are noticed.

Accurate diagnosis through blood glucose testing is essential in order to effectively manage and treat type 2 diabetes. Symptoms of type 2 diabetes can vary in terms of their presence and severity.

It is important to note that some individuals may not experience any symptoms at all, making it difficult to detect the condition. However, for those who do exhibit symptoms, they often develop gradually over time. This means that individuals may unknowingly live with type 2 diabetes for years before realizing they have the condition. If any of these symptoms are noticed, it is crucial to consult a healthcare provider for proper evaluation and diagnosis.

 Medical professionals primarily rely on blood glucose (sugar) tests to diagnose diabetes. A commonly used method is the random blood sugar test, which can be conducted at any time during the day, regardless of the last meal consumed. The normal range for random blood sugar levels is typically between 70 and 140 mg/dL (3.9 to 7.8 mmol/L).

A fasting blood sugar test is a medical procedure that involves drawing blood after a period of not consuming any food or beverages for a specific duration, typically ranging from 8 to 12 hours, often done overnight. The purpose of this test is to measure the level of glucose present in the blood after a period of fasting. A normal fasting blood sugar level is considered to be less than 100 mg/dL (5.6 mmol/L). This test is commonly used to screen for and diagnose certain medical conditions such as diabetes and prediabetes, as it provides valuable insights into the body's ability to regulate blood sugar levels.

By assessing the fasting blood sugar level, healthcare professionals can gain a better understanding of an individual's overall glucose metabolism and make informed decisions regarding their health and treatment plans if necessary. It is important to follow the recommended fasting duration before undergoing this test to ensure accurate and reliable results.

The Hemoglobin A1C test, also known as the A1C blood test, provides an indication of your average blood sugar levels over a span of two to three months. Typically, normal values for A1C fall within the range of 4 to 5.6 percent.

This test can be conducted at any time of day, regardless of whether you have eaten or not. It is a valuable tool for monitoring and managing diabetes, as it offers insight into long-term blood sugar control. By regularly monitoring your A1C levels, you can work towards maintaining optimal health and reducing the risk of complications associated with diabetes.

The oral glucose tolerance test, also known as OGTT, is a medical examination that requires the individual to consume a unique glucose solution, typically having a pleasing orange or cola flavor. The purpose of this test is to measure the levels of glucose in the blood before the consumption of the solution, as well as one and two hours after its ingestion. Due to the inconveniences associated with this procedure, such as the time it takes and the need for special glucose solution, the OGTT is not commonly utilized for testing purposes, except in the case of pregnant women.

Criteria for diagnosis refer to the specific symptoms or characteristics that must be present in order for a medical professional to identify a particular condition or illness in a patient.

These criteria are typically outlined in diagnostic manuals or guidelines, and serve as a standardized set of guidelines to ensure accurate and consistent diagnosis across healthcare settings. By carefully assessing a patient's symptoms and comparing them to the established criteria for a specific condition, healthcare providers can make an informed diagnosis and develop an appropriate treatment plan.

In some cases, multiple criteria may need to be met in order to make a definitive diagnosis, while in others, a single characteristic may be enough to confirm the presence of a particular illness.

Overall, criteria for diagnosis play a crucial role in the healthcare field by providing a framework for identifying and treating various medical conditions in a systematic and evidence-based manner.

There are specific criteria that are utilized to categorize your blood sugar levels into three different classifications: normal, increased risk, and diabetes.

Normal blood sugar levels are within the healthy range, while increased risk levels indicate higher than normal blood sugar levels that suggest a potential risk for developing diabetes in the future. On the other hand, diabetes is diagnosed when blood sugar levels consistently exceed the normal range and indicate a chronic condition that requires management and treatment. Understanding these classifications is essential for monitoring and maintaining optimal blood sugar levels for overall health and wellbeing.

A fasting blood sugar level of less than 100 mg/dL (5.6 mmol/L) is considered within the normal range and is not indicative of an elevated risk for diabetes.

Type 2 diabetes affects various major organs in the body, including the heart, blood vessels, nerves, eyes, and kidneys.

Additionally, the risk factors for diabetes are also risk factors for other serious diseases. By managing diabetes and controlling blood sugar levels, individuals can reduce their risk of developing complications and other medical conditions such as heart and blood vessel disease, nerve damage in the limbs (neuropathy), nerve damage in other areas of the body, kidney disease, and eye damage.

These complications can have significant impacts on a person's health and may require treatments such as dialysis or kidney transplants.

 Furthermore, diabetes increases the risk of developing serious eye diseases like cataracts. While the rate of progression varies, approximately 25 percent of individuals with either impaired fasting glucose or impaired glucose tolerance will develop type 2 diabetes within a period of three to five years.

If a person's test results indicate that they are at increased risk, their doctor or nurse will discuss with them the changes they can make in order to reduce their risk of developing diabetes. These changes may include improving their diet and exercise habits, losing weight, and quitting smoking if applicable. Blood sugar testing will need to be repeated annually.

Diabetes is diagnosed if a person displays one or more of the following criteria: symptoms of diabetes, along with a random blood sugar level of 200 mg/dL (11.1 mmol/L) or higher; a fasting blood sugar level of 126 mg/dL (7 mmol/L) or higher; a blood sugar level of 200 mg/dL (11.1 mmol/L) or higher two hours after an OGTT; or an A1C level of 6.5 percent (48 mmol/mol) or higher.

If diabetes is suspected based on these results, the doctor will repeat one of these tests on a different day to confirm the diagnosis. The term "increased risk" refers to individuals who have test results that indicate they are at risk of developing diabetes.

There are several categories that fall under this increased risk classification. Firstly, there is "impaired fasting glucose," which is defined as having a fasting blood sugar level between 100 and 125 mg/dL (5.6 to 6.9 mmol/L).

Secondly, there is "impaired glucose tolerance," which is defined as having a blood sugar level of 140 to 199 mg/dL (7.8 to 11 mmol/L) two hours after an oral glucose tolerance test (OGTT).

Lastly, individuals with an A1C level of 5.7 to 6.4 percent (39 to 46 mmol/mol) are also considered to be at increased risk, with the likelihood of developing type 2 diabetes being higher as the A1C levels approach the upper limit of this range.

These categories are commonly referred to as "prediabetes," and approximately one in three American adults fall into this classification. In most cases, doctors can determine whether a person has type 1 or type 2 diabetes; however, there are situations where the diagnosis is more challenging.

Type 1 diabetes is typically suspected in individuals without a strong family history of type 2 diabetes who display a combination of risk factors, such as a family history of autoimmune diseases like hypothyroidism, hyperthyroidism, or celiac sprue, along with symptoms like frequent urination and weight loss.

Furthermore, if blood sugar levels remain high even after initiating type 2 diabetes treatments, additional blood tests may be conducted to determine the specific type of diabetes.

Diabetes can have a detrimental impact on various aspects of health, including causing eye damage which can lead to conditions like cataracts and glaucoma, and potentially result in blindness.

Additionally, diabetes can increase the risk of skin problems such as bacterial and fungal infections, as well as slow the healing process of wounds which could ultimately lead to the need for amputation. Hearing impairment and obstructive sleep apnea are also common in individuals with diabetes, with obesity playing a significant role in both conditions.

 Furthermore, there is a link between type 2 diabetes and an increased risk of developing dementia, specifically Alzheimer's disease, with poor blood sugar control being associated with a faster decline in cognitive function.

Chapter 4

Prevention And Managing Of Type 2

Diabetes

The latest research on exercise regimens tailored for individuals with type 2 diabetes emphasizes the benefits of both aerobic and resistance training.

Aerobic exercises like brisk walking and cycling improve glycemic control, while resistance training helps with muscle mass and metabolic function.

Combining both types of exercise can offer comprehensive benefits for managing diabetes.

Treatment options for type 2 diabetes include lifestyle modifications, oral medications, injectable therapies, and insulin. These options are personalized based on individual needs and the progression of the condition.

It is essential to monitor blood glucose levels regularly, take medications as prescribed, and work closely with healthcare professionals to tailor a treatment plan that suits your individual needs.

Prevention of type 2 diabetes involves making healthy lifestyle choices. By eating nutritious foods, staying active, maintaining a healthy weight, and avoiding long periods of inactivity, you can reduce your risk of developing diabetes.

For those with prediabetes, metformin may be prescribed to lower the risk of progression to type 2 diabetes, especially for older adults who are obese.

Managing type 2 diabetes requires a balanced approach of healthy eating, regular exercise, monitoring blood sugar levels, and medication adherence.

It is important to focus on a well-rounded diet, limit sugary and processed foods, and engage in regular physical activity to improve insulin sensitivity and control blood sugar levels.

Chapter 5

Living well with type 2 diabetes

Building a supportive environment by educating those around you about diabetes is important. Involving your family in healthy lifestyle changes can make it a collective effort. Celebrating small victories and milestones in your diabetes management journey is important.

Living a healthy lifestyle with type 2 diabetes involves adopting a positive mindset and making sustainable choices. It is important to focus on a balanced and nutritious diet, emphasizing whole foods and portion control.

Regular physical activity should be prioritized to improve overall well-being and help manage blood sugar levels. Regularly checking your feet for any signs of complications and practicing good foot hygiene is important to prevent issues related to nerve damage.

Maintaining good oral hygiene is also crucial as diabetes can affect dental health. Being proactive in managing diabetes involves attending regular check-ups, consistently monitoring blood sugar levels, and adjusting your lifestyle accordingly.

It is important to educate yourself about diabetes and stay informed about advancements in treatment and management strategies.

Stress management techniques, such as mindfulness, meditation, or deep breathing exercises, should be incorporated into daily life as stress can have an impact on blood sugar levels.

Adequate sleep is also essential for overall health and regulating metabolism.

Lastly, it is important to stay resilient and adaptable as diabetes management may require adjustments over time. Embracing change with a positive attitude can make the process more manageable.

By prioritizing self-care, staying informed, and building a strong support network, you can lead a fulfilling life while effectively managing type 2 diabetes.

Having a support system is crucial, whether it be sharing your journey with family, friends, or joining a diabetes support group.

Open communication with healthcare professionals is also important to receive personalized advice and guidance for effective diabetes management.

Living well with type 2 diabetes is about making sustainable lifestyle choices, cultivating a positive mindset, and actively participating in your healthcare journey. Incorporating enjoyable activities into your routine, socializing, pursuing hobbies, and engaging in activities you love contribute to overall well-being.

It is important to be mindful of alcohol consumption and quit smoking if applicable, as these habits can negatively impact diabetes management.

During pregnancy, it is important to work closely with healthcare professionals to receive specialized care, closely monitor blood sugar levels, and make any necessary adjustments to medication with guidance from medical professionals to promote a healthy pregnancy.

Prior to engaging in physical activity, it is important to check your blood sugar levels. Make sure to drink plenty of water and if needed, have a snack to avoid low blood sugar levels. It is recommended to speak with healthcare professionals to create a personalized exercise regimen.

When attending social events or dining out, it's important to be proactive in making healthier choices by reviewing menus and selecting nutritious options. It's also crucial to be mindful of portion sizes and limit consumption of high-carb foods. Communicating any dietary restrictions or preferences to hosts or restaurant staff can help ensure a more enjoyable dining experience.

In terms of stress management, incorporating techniques such as mindfulness and deep breathing can be beneficial in reducing stress levels.

Additionally, establishing a consistent sleep routine can support overall well-being and help manage stress. Staying organized and managing daily tasks efficiently can also help minimize stressors in everyday life.

As individuals with type 2 diabetes age, it becomes crucial to adjust treatment plans to accommodate age-related changes.

Regular health check-ups become even more important for ongoing monitoring. Additionally, there may be considerations for potential coexisting conditions that arise.

The daily management burden of constantly monitoring blood sugar levels, medications, and dietary choices can contribute to psychological stress.

There is also the fear of potential complications, which can lead to increased anxiety and stress levels. The long-term nature of diabetes management can also contribute to feelings of depression or anxiety. The fear of experiencing hypoglycemia, or low blood sugar events, can also impact mental well-being.

Managing diabetes can also have social implications. Some individuals may experience isolation as they may withdraw socially due to fears of judgment or discomfort with managing their condition in social settings.

The impact on relationships and family dynamics may also require open communication and support. Weight management challenges can also affect body image and self-esteem, particularly in a society that often equates body weight with health.

Additionally, the use of insulin therapy and medications may lead to weight changes, which can further impact body image.

In each situation, it is essential to maintain open communication with healthcare professionals, stay proactive in self-management, and adapt strategies to the specific context in order to effectively manage type 2 diabetes.

The emotional and psychological aspects of living with type 2 diabetes can also have a significant impact. Coping with societal stereotypes and misconceptions about diabetes can be emotionally challenging, leading to feelings of stigma.

Individuals may also experience guilt and blame themselves for the development or progression of their diabetes. To cope with these emotional and psychological challenges, it can be helpful to seek educational support to better understand the condition and effective management strategies.

Additionally, professional counseling or joining support groups can provide emotional support and coping strategies for individuals with type 2 diabetes.

In the workplace, it is important to maintain open communication with colleagues about your condition and needs related to type 2 diabetes. It may also be helpful to keep healthy snacks at your desk to avoid making impulsive and unhealthy food choices. Managing stress through short breaks or relaxation techniques can also be beneficial.

Effective communication between healthcare providers and patients is essential in promoting shared decision-making, which allows individuals to feel empowered and in control of their healthcare decisions.

Regular check-ins with healthcare providers help address emotional concerns and ensure treatment plans are adjusted as needed.

 Addressing the emotional and psychological aspects of type 2 diabetes is crucial for comprehensive care, requiring collaboration among healthcare providers, mental health professionals, and support networks to improve overall well-being and quality of life.

Chapter 6

Future Directions And Research On Type 2 Diabetes

Global health initiatives are aiming to address disparities in diabetes care, particularly in low-income communities. Research into cost-effective interventions and strategies for improving healthcare access is crucial for reducing the burden of diabetes worldwide.

Future directions in the field of type 2 diabetes research are centered around advancing the options available for treatment, improving strategies for prevention, and deepening our knowledge and understanding of the disease.

The concept of personalized medicine, which involves utilizing genetic and molecular information, may offer more tailored approaches to managing diabetes.

Ongoing research is focused on exploring innovative therapies, such as the development of new medications and interventions that target the underlying mechanisms of insulin resistance. Advances in technology, such as smart insulin delivery systems and continuous glucose monitoring, aim to provide more precise and convenient tools for individuals who are managing diabetes.

Prevention of type 2 diabetes remains a critical area of investigation, with a particular emphasis on identifying risk factors and implementing effective lifestyle interventions.

Additionally, behavioral and psychosocial research seeks to better understand the impact of mental health on diabetes management and explore interventions to address these aspects.

Stem cell research is another frontier in type 2 diabetes research, with scientists investigating the potential for regenerative therapies to restore insulin-producing beta cells in the pancreas. This could revolutionize diabetes treatment by addressing the root cause of the disease.

The application of artificial intelligence and machine learning in analyzing large datasets is becoming increasingly prevalent in diabetes research. This enables researchers to gain insights into the complex nature of the disease and aids in the development of predictive models for personalized treatment plans.

Collaboration between researchers, healthcare providers, and individuals with diabetes is essential for driving progress in the field.

As technology continues to advance and our understanding of the disease deepens, the future holds promise for more effective and individualized approaches to managing and preventing type 2 diabetes.

Ultimately, the future of type 2 diabetes research involves a multidisciplinary approach, incorporating genetics, technology, behavioral science, and novel therapeutic avenues.

As these different areas of research intertwine, they have the potential to significantly impact our understanding and management of type 2 diabetes in the years to come. Exploring the role of the gut microbiome in diabetes and metabolic health is an intriguing avenue of research.

Understanding how the microbiota interacts with the body and influences metabolism could lead to novel interventions or personalized dietary recommendations.

In the realm of lifestyle interventions, research continues to optimize dietary patterns and exercise routines for diabetes management. Customizing recommendations based on individual characteristics and preferences is a key focus.

Chapter 7

Diet Recipe For Type 2 Diabetes

When it comes to managing type 2 diabetes, it is important to follow a balanced meal plan that includes a variety of nutritious foods.

One delicious option is grilled chicken breast with roasted vegetables. To prepare this meal, marinate the chicken in a mixture of olive oil, garlic, and herbs, and then grill it to perfection.

 For the roasted vegetables, choose a mix of colorful options such as broccoli, bell peppers, and carrots. Toss them in olive oil and spices, and roast them until they are tender and flavorful.

By combining these elements, you will have a tasty, low-carb option that is suitable for individuals with type 2 diabetes.

To further enhance the nutritional value of your meal, don't forget to include a leafy green salad. Choose a variety of greens such as spinach, kale, and Swiss chard, which are packed with fiber, vitamins, and minerals. Add an assortment of colorful vegetables to the salad for added nutrients. To dress the salad, make a vinaigrette using olive oil, which is a healthy fat that offers numerous benefits for individuals with diabetes.

It is important to note that individual dietary needs vary, and it is crucial to tailor your food choices to your specific health condition.

 Consulting with a healthcare professional or a registered dietitian is highly recommended to receive personalized advice and guidance based on your individual needs. They can help you create a meal plan that is suitable for your type 2 diabetes and overall health goals.

When it comes to protein, opt for lean sources such as skinless poultry, fish, tofu, and legumes. These options provide protein without excessive fat, which is important for maintaining a healthy weight and blood sugar balance.

Including healthy fats in your diet is also essential, and avocados, nuts, and olive oil are great choices. These foods contain monounsaturated fats, which can aid in blood sugar control.

In addition to the specific diet recipe mentioned above, a natural diet for type 2 diabetes often focuses on whole, unprocessed foods.

Incorporating certain food groups can be particularly beneficial for individuals with diabetes. For example, leafy greens like spinach, kale, and Swiss chard are excellent sources of fiber, vitamins, and minerals. Berries such as blueberries, strawberries, and raspberries offer a rich supply of antioxidants and are lower in sugar compared to many other fruits.

It is important to keep portion sizes in mind and avoid sugary sauces or dressings that can negatively impact blood sugar levels.

By following this balanced meal plan, you can ensure that you are providing your body with essential nutrients while managing your diabetes effectively.

Whole grains like quinoa, brown rice, and oats are preferable to refined grains for individuals with type 2 diabetes. These complex carbohydrates have a lower glycemic index, meaning they are digested more slowly and have a smaller impact on blood sugar levels. Non-starchy vegetables such as broccoli, cauliflower, zucchini, and peppers are also important additions to a diabetic-friendly diet. They are high in fiber and provide essential nutrients.

Fatty fish like salmon, mackerel, and sardines should also be included in the diet due to their high omega-3 fatty acid content.

These healthy fats have been shown to benefit heart health, which is particularly important for individuals with diabetes who may be at a higher risk of cardiovascular complications.

 Lastly, incorporating herbs and spices like cinnamon, turmeric, and garlic can have positive effects on blood sugar levels.

To complement the dish, consider adding a side of quinoa or brown rice. Both of these whole grains are high in fiber, which can help manage blood sugar levels.

They also have a lower glycemic index compared to refined grains, meaning they have a smaller impact on blood sugar. Including these grains in your meal will not only provide essential nutrients but also contribute to a balanced and diabetic-friendly approach.

Acknowledgement

I wish to thank Almighty God for the inspiration to undertake this project and contribute to the society positively.

About the Author

Leo Chambers is a creative writer and Digital Content Creator.